Extracts from the
Haynes

Brain
Manual

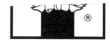

Dr. Ian Banks

Contents

© Ian Banks 2011
Revision due October 2013

(066 - 12549)

ISBN: 978 0 85761 028 7

The Author and the Publisher have taken care to ensure that the advice given in this edition is current at the time of publication. The Reader is advised to read and understand the instructions and information material included with all medicines recommended, and to consider carefully the appropriateness of any treatments. The Author and the Publisher will have no liability for adverse results, inappropriate or excessive use of the remedies offered in this book or their level of effectiveness in individual cases. The Author and the Publisher do not intend that this book be used as a substitute for medical advice. Advice from a medical practitioner should always be sought for any symptom or illness.

Printed in the UK.
Haynes Publishing, Sparkford, Yeovil, Somerset BA22 7JJ, England
Haynes North America, Inc, 861 Lawrence Drive, Newbury Park, California 91320, USA
Haynes Publishing Nordiska AB, Box 1504, 751 45 UPPSALA, Sweden

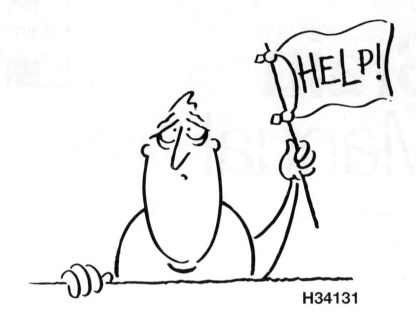

H34131

Introduction

1 Just as our physical health is linked to our genes and our lifestyle, so too is our mental health. For instance, through their genes, some people may be more susceptible to anxiety or depression. Others may develop a mental health problem as a result of child abuse, substance misuse or experiencing a traumatic event. All of us are vulnerable when it comes to major life changes – a death in the family, divorce or losing our job. Even positive changes, such as having a new baby or moving house, can be stressful and have a negative impact on our mental well-being.

2 Experiencing a mental health problem should not be a cause of shame any more than having pneumonia or breaking a leg. In fact, mental health problems are extremely common. Indeed, 1 in 4 of us will experience one at some point in our lives.

3 Although mental health problems affect both men and women, men are much less likely to seek help from their doctor. Men traditionally expect themselves to be competitive and successful, tough and self-reliant. They can find it very difficult to admit that they are feeling fragile and vulnerable. If they do see their doctor, they are more likely to talk about their physical symptoms than the emotional and psychological ones. As a result, many men do not get the help they need and make their problems worse by abusing alcohol and drugs.

4 Mental health problems include a wide range of conditions. Some affect our sense of well-being, such as anxiety and mild depression. Other mental health problems can be more severe, such as schizophrenia, where a person can at times lose contact with reality.

5 Many mental health problems respond very well to treatment, so it is important to seek professional help. If you are feeling wretched, don't hold back – talk to your GP, a family member or friend.

Stress and work

1 There is a lot of rubbish written about stress and much misconception stems from the word being poorly defined and meaning different things to different people!

2 In a nutshell stress is the response we feel when things that are happening exceed our ability to cope.

3 Unfortunately stress is often confused with every day pressure – which we all experience on a regular basis! In fact we actually need pressure to perform at our best. Think of an actor or an athlete – the pressure they feel before they perform helps them give a good performance and this is the same for any of us – think of positive examples of pressure helping you give your best!

4 Problems, however, arise when the amount of pressure we experience becomes too great. This may be due to one major event such as a bereavement, or an accumulation of many smaller hassles one after the other without enabling time to recover. The curve illustrates what happens.

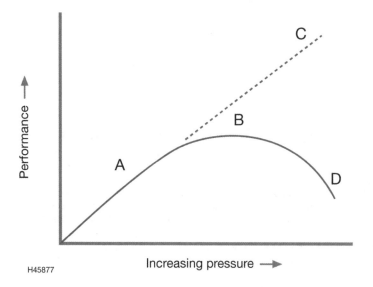

H45877

5 As pressure increases so does our performance (A) until we eventually reach our peak (B). Give us more and more pressure beyond or peak and we think we carry on being more and more productive (C). However, in actual fact we do not. We actually start to show adverse reactions or stress. At first we may just be irritable or snappy; make silly mistakes and be unable think clearly. However, If the pressure continues this becomes worse, our performance drops and we can start to exhibit a variety of physical symptoms (D). We can also show mental symptoms such as anxiety and eventually depression.

6 Stress is therefore not a medical condition, but if it is prolonged or not corrected then illness can arise, and this is why it is important to recognise stress and to have some simple tools for dealing with the issues that can create it.

7 We are all different (thank goodness!), and there is much variation in our capacity to cope with the very many different things that happen to us in daily life. We therefore need to be aware that stress is not a sign of weakness but simply reflects overload at a given time.

8 The signs of stress may be anywhere in the body from head to toe and can be very variable from one person to the next. Headaches, palpitations, upset stomach, sweating, strange behaviour and many others symptoms can occur when stress arises and many consultations with doctors complaining of aches or pains or other ailments are the physical manifestations of the brain complaining it can't cope!

9 If a computer gets overloaded – ultimately it may 'lock' or 'crash', people are the same, and a serious stress related illness can be thought of as the human version of an overloaded processor!

> There are many definitions of stress, but perhaps the best is that adopted by the Health and Safety Executive who define stress as:
> 'An adverse reaction a person has to excessive pressures or other types of demands placed upon them'.

So why does too much pressure turn to stress ?

10 To answer this question it is necessary to understand something called the stress response.

11 This is an adaptive response which evolved to help our ancestors cope with physical threats such as being chased by a woolly mammoth. This response, often termed the 'fight or flight' response, comprises physiological changes in our body that result in both mental and physical alertness. The stress response is mainly caused by the release of adrenalin and noradrenalin which alongside many other changes in the body result in the common symptoms of dry mouth, sweaty palms, elevated heart rate, butterflies in the tummy.

12 Just imagine a large lion has just walked in to the room behind you – unless you are a professional lion tamer (and maybe even if you are!), the body reaction described above is quite recognisable and may even include some looseness of the bowels.

13 You may recognise these symptoms as 'nerves' before a job interview or an examination.

14 The major changes during the stress response are outlined in the following table.

- Increase in sensitivity of nervous system – increases speed with which we may react to a threat.
- Muscles tense ready for action.
- Breathing rate increases – to take in more oxygen into the lungs. This is then carried by the blood to the muscles where it combines with glucose to make energy.
- More glucose is released from the liver and into the blood stream – used for increased energy.
- Heart rate and blood pressure increase – blood carrying oxygen and sugar is pumped to the muscles to make energy.
- Sweating increases – to cool body down during running or fighting.
- Digestive system slows down – if fighting for survival don't need to be digesting food, energy is therefore conserved.

● Reproductive system slows down – not necessary if you are fighting for survival! So energy is also conserved here.

● Another hormone, cortisol, is released.

Additional effects of cortisol

15 One of the main functions of cortisol is to regulate the metabolism. During stress it enables the body to produce more glucose to keep it going longer. A by product of this is the production of fatty acids which can result in increased production of cholesterol. Increased cholesterol affects the cardiovascular system.

16 Cortisol also dampens down the immune system so over time we become more susceptible to infections.

17 While the stress response is still useful for occasional modern day physical threats, such as being chased by an attacker or by a lion on safari, most of our modern day pressures are not physical and therefore do not merit a physical response.

18 Many are also generated from work. For example:

● The difficult boss.

● Too much work.

● E-mails.

● Angry customers.

19 We cannot respond to these by running away or fighting so we sit and bottle it up. We therefore do not do what the stress response is gearing us up to do. Added to this is the fact that one pressure comes immediately after another. We do not have time to get the physiological changes out of our system before the next pressure comes along.

We can cause our own stress by our thoughts and fears

20 We are afraid of not being good enough or looking stupid. Fear of job security is now also very common. Pressures like these never really go away, but are constantly generating the response. Instead of being helpful, the changes taking place in our body start to work against us and we start to suffer from stress symptoms.

Where to get help

21 Many larger businesses rely on their occupational health departments to provide advice, support and help. Workers in smaller businesses may get help through their unions, NHS Direct or via the Health and Safety Executive who have their own occupational health experts.

22 Many organisations have an Employee Assistance Programme (EAP) or some kind of counselling service. If so give them a ring. The service is always totally confidential.

23 As an individual there are also many sources of help available. Your GP may be a first port of call or contact one of the many organisations contributing to this book. They are all there to help.

24 Do not be put off seeking help by the perceived stigma. As has been said many times, stress is not a weakness, it is basically just overload which can happen to anybody. Often it is the really good people who give 200% that suffer. Surely it is better to recognise a problem and try to fix it before it becomes worse than refuse to address it until it becomes so bad you cause others stress by going off sick.

25 Addressing an issue of stress is not a weakness, it is a strength!

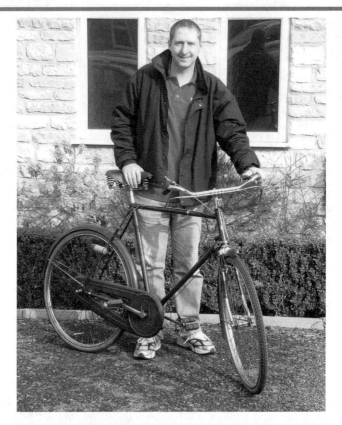

So what should we do to reduce the effects of stress?

- Identify causes – only then can you tackle the issues.

- Change your behaviour to reduce the onset of the stress response, eg avoid unnecessary conflict; learn to be more assertive; don't procrastinate; attend a stress management course. If the stress is work related, raise the issue with your manager. Employers now have a legal duty of care to do what is reasonably practicable to ensure staff do not suffer from work related stress. If your manager knows you have a work related problem they must try to help reduce it.

- Change perceptions – look at different ways you can see things. You are not indispensable, things do not have to always be perfect. Talk things over with a friend or colleague: this will often help you change your perceptions

- Make sure you take regular breaks to allow your body time to recover between pressures.

- Learn to relax – relaxation helps reduce the stress response and hence the detrimental effect.

- Exercise – this helps you reduce the effects of stress. That is what the caveman did. Through exercise you are doing what the stress response geared you up to do.

26 Most of all you must realise that stress is not a weakness. Given the right combination of events, stress can happen to anybody.

27 If you experience stress take action to reduce it before it gets too serious. Managing stress is about taking responsibility for yourself. Nobody else can do it for you.

Physical activity

1 Exercise is not just good for the heart, it is also good for the mind. Just as pumping iron makes you stronger and able to lift heavier loads, taking regular exercise enables your brain to cope better when things get stressful. The fitter your body, the more reserves you

> Walking is man's best medicine
> Hippocrates,
> Ancient Greek Physician

have to draw on when under pressure. The same applies for the brain.

2 Scientists have shown that people who take regular physical activity are less likely to suffer from depression and anxiety, and are better able to cope with stress. Studies have found that exercise can be as effective as anti-depressant drugs in cases of mild or moderate depression. More evidence on just how exercise affects the brain is emerging all the time. The latest research suggests that fitter people have better cognitive functioning. This means they are better at remembering things, planning, organising and juggling different tasks. Also, regular physical activity can help some of the mental decline that is associated with ageing. Being physically active is part of the routine maintenance for a healthy brain.

> One survey found that 85 per cent of people with mental health problems who had tried exercise found it helpful. Unlike anti-depressants, people say that exercise feels like a 'natural' way to respond to feeling down – it gives people a sense of achievement and control which can help counter feelings of hopelessness.
>
> Mental Health Foundation

3 Both exercise and physical activity are good for mental health. Just going out for a stroll can improve mental well-being, so you don't have to be a fitness fanatic to benefit. Generally, the more exercise you do, the better it is for preventing depression.

Operating systems – how exercise improves mental health

4 During exercise, our brains release chemicals similar to morphine called endorphins. These are sometimes called feel-good hormones and are important in regulating emotion and pain perception. Anti-depressants produced by drug companies are designed to improve the balance of these brain chemicals. It is likely that exercise does this naturally and therefore leads to improved mood and feelings of well-being.

5 Another theory is referred to as the thermogenic hypothesis. Exercise increases the body temperature, which in turn leads to reduced muscle tension and feelings of relaxation and well-being. The Scandinavians obviously think this is true judging by their love of saunas!

6 Exercise provides us with 'time out' and takes our mind off anxious or stressful thoughts. But exercise can also boost our self-esteem by making us feel more confident by completing an activity, doing something worthwhile or accomplishing a challenge, whether it is marathon or simply a walk to the top of a hill.

7 Physical activity gives us something positive to focus on and aim for and provides opportunities to meet new people. This stops us from feeling isolated and unsupported.

Rebooting the system

8 Have you ever watched a toddler at play? They stand up, sit down, run around, gyrate and contort their little bodies into all sorts of positions. This activity is vital for their development and their health. As we get older, we lose much of that natural physical activity as life's demands get the better of us. By the time

we reach our teens, very few of us actually still do enough exercise to benefit our health. We need to make a special effort to build activity back into our lives, especially as technology seems hell-bent on removing every opportunity to be active by giving us cars, computers, escalators, power tools and remote controls.

9 The Government has come up with guidelines, based on years of research, about the minimum amount of physical activity we should be doing. These guidelines state that, to maintain good health, we should aim to be active at a moderate intensity for thirty minutes, at least five times a week. Only about 30% of the UK population meet the current Government guidelines and 6 out of 10 men currently don't do enough physical activity to benefit their health. Most people believe that they are active enough and describe themselves as 'fit', but the statistics tell a different story.

10 Researchers are unclear about the amount of activity needed to maintain a healthy mind, but the evidence suggests that 30 minutes, five times a week at a moderate intensity is also the level of physical activity needed to improve mental health.

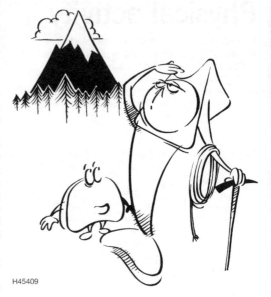

H45409

Where do I start?

11 Exercise is good for you whatever your mental state. It is the oil that lubricates a healthy mind and

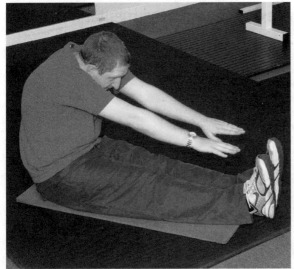

keeps it healthy. It can also help as a remedy when things aren't so good. If you're feeling down, then exercise may be the last thing on your mind and starting an exercise programme can be challenging. That's why it is important to start gently and build up gradually and choose something that is manageable and fun.

12 It is a good idea to check with your doctor before you increase the amount of physical activity that you do or before starting an exercise programme. Take a look at the questions below. If you have answered 'yes' to one or more of them, then discuss your plans with your doctor before you start.

13 This questionnaire is designed to help you decide whether you are physically ready to take up more exercise. Answering 'yes' to any of these questions does not necessarily mean that you cannot become more active, but you may need to check with your doctor so that he or she can help you structure a safe and effective programme.

- Has your doctor ever said that you have a heart condition or have you ever experienced a stroke or blood clot?

- Do you ever experience pain in your chest when you are physically active or at any other time?

- Do you ever feel faint, lose your balance or lose consciousness?

- Do you have a bone or joint condition such as rheumatoid arthritis?

- Is your doctor currently prescribing medication for high blood pressure or a heart condition?

- Have you had surgery in the last three months?

- Do you suffer from epilepsy that is hard to control?

- Do you suffer from diabetes?

> Moderate intensity activity is described as any exercise that uses the large muscle groups (such as walking, dancing, sport, gardening, cycling) and makes you breathe slightly deeper and feel slightly warmer.

> By feeling and gradually looking fitter and healthier, physical activity leads to a more positive body image and boosts self-confidence and self-esteem.

14 It is very unlikely that your doctor will tell you that you cannot increase your activity level. Very few conditions are made worse with exercise. In fact most physical and mental conditions are improved with regular physical activity. The main thing is to choose the right exercise for your level of fitness and ability and build up gradually.

Is it safe?

15 Very few conditions do not benefit from regular physical activity or exercise. In fact, not becoming more active is likely to be much more detrimental to your health. Choose gentle activities such as walking to get you started and seek out professional help if you are trying something new like a gym or a new sport.

> Physical activity makes you sleep better. Lack of sleep (or poor quality sleep) is a problem that is commonly associated with depression. Becoming more active can therefore help with this condition.

16 It is quite natural to feel hot and sweaty during exercise and to be breathing much more heavily. This is usually a sign that you are working at the correct intensity. However, experiencing any of the 'Stop Signs' should act as a warning that you may be overdoing things.

17 Many GPs can 'prescribe' exercise for patients, referring them to schemes where they will be helped to develop their own personal exercise programme under the supervision of a qualified trainer. Not every doctor's surgery can offer this service, but it is worth finding out from your doctor whether such a scheme is available in your area and whether it is suitable for you.

STOP SIGNS

Palpitations

A fast or irregular heartbeat is a danger signal.

Pain or discomfort

Expect to feel a little discomfort at first, especially if you are unused to physical activity, but any pain in the chest or upper body, particularly the left arm, is a sign to stop exercising and seek your doctor's advice.

Breathlessness

If you are finding it hard to control your breathing or gasping for breath and this does not subside as you decrease the intensity of your physical activity, stop and consult your doctor.

Fainting

If you faint during or just after exercise, seek your doctor's advice before continuing. If you experience dizziness or nausea during exercise, slow down and wait to see if it subsides. If it does not, then stop the activity.

Tips for fitting exercise into your day

Write your exercise sessions into your diary as you would any other appointment. Remember that this time spent on physical activity is just as important as other commitments.

Get up earlier

Go for a walk or an early gym session. Research has shown that people who exercise in the morning are more likely to stick with it. It is often easy to find excuses not to exercise as the day progresses and fills with unforeseen demands on your time.

Do the housework and make it count

Vigorous sweeping, mopping or scrubbing are all excellent forms of exercise. You'll also get the pleasure of a clean home and a happy family.

Take the kids out for a walk or a game of football

Kids need exercise too!

Get off the train or bus a stop earlier and walk the last part of your journey to work

If there is a lot of traffic, it may even prove to be quicker than the motorised option.

Take the stairs instead of the lift or escalator

Remember every little bit counts and it all adds up.

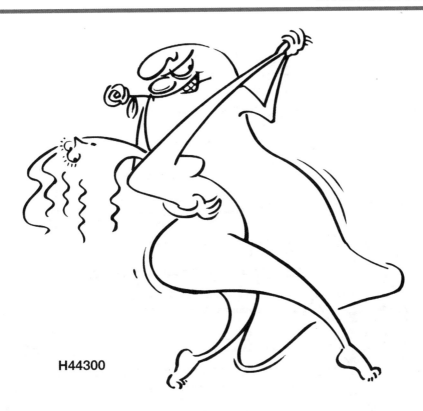

H44300

What physical activity should I choose?

18 If you don't fancy the idea of joining a gym, there are plenty of other ways of becoming more active and getting more exercise. Many people who start on a physical activity or exercise programme give up within a matter of months. Usually this is because they have chosen activities that are unmanageable, either because they make too many demands on their time, or because they are too strenuous. Physical activity shouldn't feel like hard work, it should be fun and enjoyable. Aim to include lots of variety in your exercise programme, combining daily walks or cycle rides with weekly sporting activities like football or fencing. You could also try more adventurous activities like kayaking or orienteering.

Seasonal Affective Disorder (SAD) is a type of winter depression that affects an estimated 1/2 million people every winter in the UK, particularly between September and April. Although it can be treated with light therapy and drugs, just getting out in daylight hours can help many people. Exercising outdoors, particularly at lunchtime during the winter, can help counteract the effects of SAD.

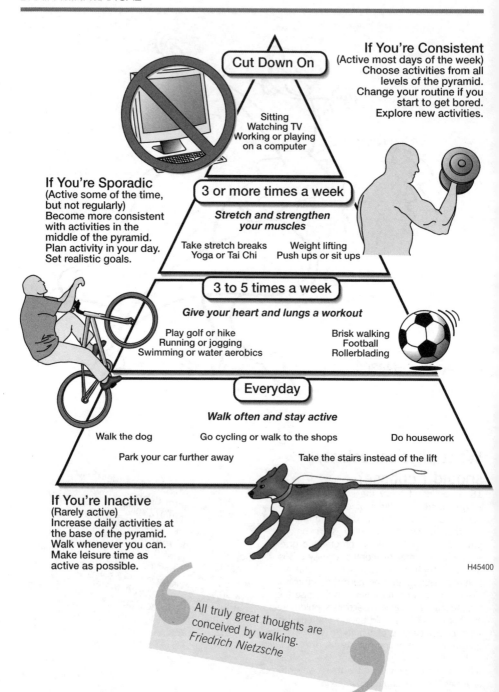

Cut Down On

Sitting
Watching TV
Working or playing
on a computer

If You're Consistent
(Active most days of the week)
Choose activities from all
levels of the pyramid.
Change your routine if you
start to get bored.
Explore new activities.

If You're Sporadic
(Active some of the time,
but not regularly)
Become more consistent
with activities in the
middle of the pyramid.
Plan activity in your day.
Set realistic goals.

3 or more times a week

*Stretch and strengthen
your muscles*

Take stretch breaks
Yoga or Tai Chi

Weight lifting
Push ups or sit ups

3 to 5 times a week

Give your heart and lungs a workout

Play golf or hike
Running or jogging
Swimming or water aerobics

Brisk walking
Football
Rollerblading

Everyday

Walk often and stay active

Walk the dog   Go cycling or walk to the shops   Do housework

Park your car further away   Take the stairs instead of the lift

If You're Inactive
(Rarely active)
Increase daily activities at
the base of the pyramid.
Walk whenever you can.
Make leisure time as
active as possible.

H45400

All truly great thoughts are
conceived by walking.
Friedrich Nietzsche

Mental activity

Research by scientist Robert S. Wilson and his colleagues in Chicago showed that nuns, monks and priests aged over 65 who were most mentally active – reading, doing crosswords and games, visiting museums and so on – had a roughly 50 per cent lower risk of developing Alzheimer's disease over a four and a half year period than those who were least mentally active.

1 How many times have you heard the phrase 'You know... my memory just isn't what it used to be?' One of the reasons our memories let us down as we get older is that we may have got out of the habit of learning new things, and the brain may have become inactive through lack of use.

2 Being more mentally sharp and increasing mental activity can help counter some of the more negative effects that ageing can have on the brain and keep you more mentally fit as you get older. As a result of this you can get more pleasure out of life.

Learning

3 Many of us do much of our learning in the first three decades of our lives but learn relatively few new skills in the subsequent five decades. Acquiring new learning and new information at any age is a good way to revive brain cells.

4 One reason that some people are less sharp when they are over 50 is that they don't bother to learn as much as they did when they were younger, and, contrary to popular belief, provided physical health is retained, there is little evidence that mental ability declines significantly until extreme old age.

5 Many older people surprise themselves by the pleasure and satisfaction they get improving their early education, learning a topic that has long interested them, such as a new language, coming to terms with modern technology or just broadening their mental horizons.

6 Your local library should be able to help you with personal study or research and your local authority education office is responsible for providing adult education classes, usually with concessionary rates for older people.

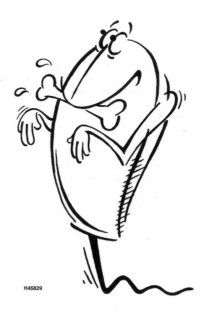

H45829

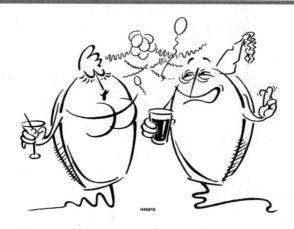

New Technology

7 There is positive evidence that use of new technologies such as the Internet and e-mail can promote mental health in later life. Older men can create and sustain social networks, learning new skills and maintaining contact with family members, many of whom may be geographically dispersed.

Social networks

8 Human beings are highly social animals and interacting with other people is important to keep our brains active and stimulated. Unfortunately men are less likely to discuss how they feel with other men and don't have the same degree of intimate relationships that women do.

9 Throughout most of our lives we are continually developing relationships with other people – family members, friends, the wider community and work colleagues. Many older men, despite possible ill-health or regardless of the transitions they experience in their lives, have been able to develop and maintain old and new relationships in a variety of ways. Taking up a hobby, a social activity or travel allows older people to revive friendships and make new friends.

Spirituality

10 Evidence points to the positive influence of spirituality and religious belief on mental health needs in later life. Benefits include a sense of purpose, inclusion in social support networks and even a sense of coming to terms with mortality.

Arts and Health

11 The link between arts and health has long been known: over 2,000 years ago, Apollo was the Greek god of medicine and fine arts.

12 The range of art forms is very diverse and can include painting, drawing, photography, pottery, drama, dance, music and film-making. Even within these art forms there are many ways to become involved; 'music', for example, can offer opportunities to listen to music, go to a concert, sing, play musical instruments or mount a full-scale orchestral production.

> Everyone is creative... imagination, innovation and original expression are vital components of what it is to be human and to be part of society.
>
> *Culture and Creativity: The Next Ten Years, Department for Culture, Media and Sport.*

Feed your head!

1 The word diet may conjure up images of sparse portions and grumbling hunger pangs. However in this context the word 'diet' means what you eat rather than how you can lose weight. Nutrition and diet are important factors in any health programme. Older men may become overweight or may have been eating incorrectly – either type of eating behaviour can be affected by poor memory.

> Rats fed on the equivalent of burger and chips show poorer memory and mental agility compared with rats that are fed on a less fatty diet

2 The good news is that a lot of benefit can be gained by making minor changes. Introducing plenty of fruit and vegetables and foods that are high in fibre and low in sugar, salt and fat can help to increase energy and alertness. For example fish, vegetables and fruit – particularly dark fruit such as cranberries and blackcurrants – are good for a healthy brain. Eat lots of them as part of a balanced diet and you will be doing your brain a favour.

3 Foods high in saturated fats – such as crisps, ready made meals and processed food – dull your mental faculties and should be eaten only in moderation.

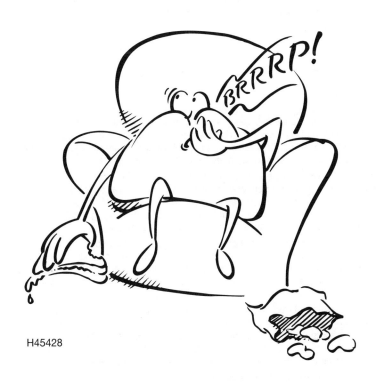

H45428

Sexuality

1 Men in general, and young men in particular, may face a wide range of pressures and difficulties around relationships with men and women. It is normal for all men to find sexuality confusing at various times in their lives – and not only when younger.

2 There are no simple answers to the question of sexuality. It is a lively, changing, powerful and life-affirming force. What we like to do, where, when, how and who with are complex questions of individual taste and choice.

3 Some men may feel they should be having a certain amount of sex, and that any less (or more) is unacceptable. Men may often have anxieties about their relationships to women, or to other men. There are many moral, rules and judgments around sex, but only one answer: **so long as the people involved have freely consented, there should be no moral judgement.**

- It's OK to be straight, and
- It's OK to be bisexual, and
- It's OK to be gay, and
- It's OK to change your mind.

4 However, life can be more complicated in practice. People may have had heterosexual experiences or relationships first. Might have been involved in a long-term heterosexual relationship, perhaps got married and had children, and then become interested in someone of the same sex. Or people might have been having gay relationships in secret. This can leave people feeling torn or confused. This experience is very common, given the pressure in our society for everyone to be heterosexual.

5 Being heterosexual is so completely taken for granted in our society, even now, that most people just assume they are going to grow up heterosexual and stay that way. Falling in love with someone of the same sex, or being turned on by them, can be inspiring – but also frightening, because being lesbian, gay or bisexual is not yet generally acceptable. People can that tell us it's wrong – and that can make it even more difficult for individuals who want to talk things over with someone.

6 An important first step is to be able to be honest with yourself about your feelings. It might take time to realise whether you are feeling an effect of difficulties in your heterosexual relationships, or whether having lesbian or gay, or bisexual, relationships is what suits you best. It might feel like a big step to take, but talking to someone will help you sort out your feelings and it might be a huge relief to talk to someone.

7 You might feel relatively relaxed about these issues, or you might feel revulsion and dislike. If you do feel able to admit an attraction, it can bring on feelings of self-hatred, as a result of society's rejection of homosexuality. But it's important to remember that there are many ways of being a man and the standard idea is generally too narrow. It might take a while to become more comfortable with a more modern sense of sexuality and masculinity, but talking about your feelings with someone you trust will help.

8 Many people find counselling or therapy very helpful.

9 See the *Contacts* Section for organisations that will understand and can help.